Corporate Wellness

Office-friendly Exercises and Metabolism-boosting Foods

Table of Contents

Chapter 1. Introduction

Welcome to a Special Report that is set to transform your working days into a journey to holistic wellness! Our focus? "Corporate Wellness: Office-friendly Exercises and Metabolism-boosting Foods." Whether you're spending long hours at the office or working remotely at home, this vibrant and inspiring guide will help you incorporate healthy habits into your daily routine, making you feel brighter, more energetic, and significantly improving your productivity. Discover simple yet effective exercises adapted for your work setting and delicious indulgences that not only tickle your taste buds, but also rev up your metabolism. Who knew staying fit and healthy could be so delightful and seamlessly fit into your corporate life? Let's embark on this wellness journey together and turn your 'busy' into 'active' and 'healthy'! This report is more than just reading material; it's an investment in your wellbeing. Will you join us for this exciting voyage?

Chapter 2. Understanding Corporate Wellness: An Overview

Corporate wellness, a term increasingly heard in halls of modern enterprises, refers to the physical and mental health, as well as the overall wellbeing of the employees in an organization. It involves practices and activities that a company may hold as an initiative to support better health for its employees. The objective is not only to create a much healthier and happier workforce but also to improve productivity, increase staff retention, reduce absenteeism, and create a positive company culture enriched with wellness.

2.1. The Concept Behind Corporate Wellness

In the fast-paced business environment, companies often push their resources, technology, and most importantly, their personnel to the limit to stay competitive. But the exponential growth of the corporate sector has seen an equally dramatic rise in work-related stress, sedentary lifestyle diseases and overall health issues amongst the working population. This situation brought to light the need for a comprehensive approach to maintain and improve employee health - giving rise to the concept of corporate wellness.

Corporate wellness is a holistic approach, taking into consideration not just the physical but also emotional, intellectual, and even financial health of employees. It underscores the idea that fostering healthy habits and positive lifestyle changes has a direct impact on an employees' productivity and, consequently, the company's success.

2.2. The Impact of Corporate Wellness

Let's delve deeper into how corporate wellness impacts the employees and the organization:

Health Benefits: Corporate wellness initiatives induce employees to adopt healthier lifestyles, hence mitigating issues related to sedentary work like obesity, hypertension, diabetes, and an array of musculoskeletal disorders.

Productivity Boost: With better physical health comes improved mental health, both of which contribute to increased productivity. A healthier and happier employee is an efficient, creative, and motivated one, sparking more innovation.

Reduction in Absenteeism: Wellness programs can help decrease absenteeism. Healthier employees are less likely to fall sick, reducing sick leaves and increasing the overall operating efficiency of an organization.

Increased Employee Retention: Wellness programs create a supportive and caring environment, making employees feel valued. This sense of being cared for promotes loyalty and job satisfaction, leading to increased employee retention.

Kick-start for a Healthy Culture: Wellness doesn't stop at the workplace. Healthy habits picked up at work are carried back home. An organization that emphasizes wellness fosters not just physically and mentally fit employees, but also, by extension, healthier families and communities.

2.3. Corporate Wellness Programs: The Building Blocks

Now that we've taken a closer look at what corporate wellness includes and its impact on the organization and its members let's explore the building blocks of an effective corporate wellness program.

Health Assessments and Screenings: These are the tools that help identify potential health risks and provide a clear picture of the overall health status of your team. This information is vital to design an effective program tailored to your employees' needs.

Physical Activity Programs: These can range from lunchtime yoga classes to inter-departmental sports competitions. The goal is to engage employees in a physical activity they enjoy, thereby reducing stress and boosting overall health.

Nutritional Activities: Office competitions involving cooking, having a salad bar, or regular sessions with a nutritionist are some ways to encourage healthy eating habits.

Mental Health Initiatives: Stress management workshops, meditation classes, or mental health days off can help employees better manage stress.

Health Education: Seminars, newsletters, and workshops to educate employees about wellness, disease prevention, and healthy lifestyles can be a major game-changer in long-term health management.

Challenges and Incentives: Creating a competitive environment through challenges and rewards can motivate employees to stay committed to the wellness program.

2.4. The Role of Technology in Corporate Wellness

In corporate wellness, technology serves as a cornerstone to effectively engage employees, track progress and measure the success of wellness programs. From step trackers and wellness apps to telemedicine and wearable technology, companies are leveraging digital platforms to boost health initiatives.

Mobile applications make it easy for employees to manage and monitor their health, participate in wellness challenges, connect with health coaches, and access a wealth of informative content related to nutrition, exercise, mental health, and more.

Telemedicine is a significant technological leap in corporate wellness, providing employees with immediate access to healthcare services irrespective of their location.

Wearable technology aids in personalized health monitoring by providing data about sleep patterns, heart rate, activity levels, etc., encouraging employees to stay active and hit their health goals.

2.5. Corporate Wellness: Embarking on a Journey of Transformation

Companies are increasingly recognizing the undeniable link between employee wellness and business success. As such, corporate wellness is no longer perceived as an expense but an investment that yields compelling returns in the shape of healthier, happier, and more productive employees.

Engaging in corporate wellness goes beyond mere programs; it is about creating a culture of overall wellbeing. It's about cultivating an environment where employees can work, grow, and thrive—physically, mentally, and emotionally. A holistic approach to health and wellness paves the way for a resilient, motivated, and high-performance workforce, creating a successful, vibrant business.

The journey towards corporate wellness is a marathon, not a sprint. It's not just about launching a program; it's a ripple effect, augmenting health and happiness amongst employees, boosting their productivity, and improving the overall success of the developing world of business. Embarking on this journey is an enlightening process that draws attention to the role of health in a professional's life and inspires a transformation journey towards a healthier and more satisfying life.

Implementing a robust corporate wellness strategy might seem like a huge undertaking initially, but the potential outcomes in the form of improved employee wellbeing and enhanced organizational strength are well worth the effort. Its impact stretches out in ripples, touching the employee, their families, the organization, and the community. Incorporating wellness at a corporate level is the first significant stride toward a healthier future, laying the foundation for a healthier, happier, and more productive work environment.

So, here's to embracing corporate wellness, the secret ingredient to a vibrant and thriving corporate culture!

Chapter 3. Decoding Metabolism: The Magic Within

Often, when we think about health and wellness, we focus solely on exercise and diet. However, there's a hidden hero that plays a significant role in maintaining our well-being: metabolism. Today, we'll explore the fascinating world of metabolism, understand its functions and nuances, and learn how we can enhance it naturally through our everyday habits.

3.1. Understanding Metabolism

Metabolism, while often described as a singular function, is actually a collection of chemical reactions that occur within our bodies, crucial for life. These reactions transform the fuel in the food we eat into energy required to power everything we do, from moving to thinking to growing. Simply put, Metabolism is our bodies best-kept secret power!

Broadly, metabolism can be categorized into two types: Anabolism, which uses energy to build components of cells, and Catabolism, which breaks down organic matter to harvest energy. A well-balanced interaction between these two processes is what keeps us ticking.

3.2. Factors Affecting Metabolism

Several aspects determine how our body metabolizes nutrients. These include:

- Your age: As we age, our metabolic rate generally slows down.

- Your sex: Men typically have a higher metabolism than women because they tend to have more muscle mass.

- Your body composition: The more muscle and less fat you have, the higher your metabolic rate.

- Environmental factors: Weather, stress, and other external elements can influence metabolism.

- Exercise: Physical activity can boost your metabolic rate.

- Hormonal factors: Thyroid and other hormones can impact how quickly or slowly our body metabolizes food.

3.3. The Metabolism-Energy Connection

A lot of circumstances we go through daily, often without much thought, are powered by metabolism. The heat we generate that keeps us warm on a cold day, the energy that propels us up a flight of stairs, the power behind our thoughts and emotions, even the growth and repair of cells, are all manifestations of metabolic processes.

The food we eat is metabolized into energy that can be immediately used or, when in excess, stored for future use. This stored energy is typically in the form of fat, hence why when we eat more calories than we burn, weight gain ensues.

3.4. Feeding Your Metabolism

But how do we regulate our metabolism? Is it something we're stuck with for life, or can we change it? The good news is, through certain foods and behaviors, we can potentially increase our metabolic rate, aid weight loss, and increase overall wellness.

Here are few tips:

- Don't skip meals: Skipping meals may cause your body to go into a fat-storing starvation mode, slowing down your metabolism as a survival mechanism.

- Eat enough proteins, which are generally harder for the body to break down, increasing calorie burning during digestion (also known as the thermogenic effect).

- Drink plenty of water: This keeps your organs functioning at their best, which helps maintain a healthy metabolic rate. It's especially effective cold, as your body burns calories warming it up.

- Spice up your food: Capsaicin, a compound found in peppers, may boost metabolism.

- Consume small meals throughout the day: This keeps your metabolism active.

3.5. Moving for Metabolism

Physical activity is another vital factor that influences your metabolism. Regular exercise isn't just about burning calories; it's about tuning your metabolism to function swiftly and efficiently even when you're at rest. Here are some ways to incorporate more movements into your day:

- Take short breaks to move around: Prolonged sitting can lead to slow metabolic rate and fat storage. Standing, stretching, or walking even for a few minutes can aid in keeping your metabolism active.

- Incorporate strength training into your workout regime: It helps build lean muscle mass, which can boost your metabolism.

- Consider high-intensity interval training (HIIT) workouts: These exercises can rev up your metabolism and keep it elevated for hours after your workout.

- Small movements count: Remember, every bit of movement helps. Even fidgeting has been shown to increase energy expenditure and metabolism!

In the end, the miracle of metabolism comes down to balance – consuming the right foods, maintaining an active lifestyle, combined with knowledge about your own body's workings, can offer a solid foundation for a healthier, happier life at home and within your corporate world. Understanding and supporting your metabolism is an essential step to better wellbeing. A well-nourished and well-moved body is a powerhouse of energy and positivity, ready to ace professional challenges and personal goals alike.

Chapter 4. Conquer the Chair: Office-friendly Exercises

Whether you're a high-powered CEO or an enthusiastic start-up entrepreneur, office work typically involves long hours of sitting in front of a computer. This sedentary lifestyle can potentially lead to a slew of health issues, including obesity, heart disease, and more. However, with an active approach to your daily routine, you can avoid these risks without disrupting your professional commitments. This chapter delves into various exercises that you can perform right within the confines of your office space.

4.1. Warm-up and Stretching

Before plunging into any exercise routine, it's essential to prepare your body for the movements to come. Warm-up exercises not only boost circulation and enhance muscle performance, but also decrease the risk of injuries.

1. Neck Rolls: Sit tall in your chair. Slowly tilt your head towards your right shoulder and roll it down towards your chest and to the left. Repeat this circular motion five times, then switch directions.

2. Shoulder Rolls: While sitting up straight, roll your shoulders up towards your ears, then back and down. Completing this circle five times one way, then reversing will help ease any tension accumulated from long hours of working.

3. Wrist Circles: Extend your arms in front of you and slowly rotate your wrists in a circular motion. Do ten circles clockwise and ten counter clockwise.

4.2. Strength and Cardio Workouts

Beyond stretching, it's crucial to incorporate strength and cardio activities into your office routine. These will not only help maintain muscle mass and heart health but also improve your focus and energy at work.

1. Chair Squats: Stand in front of your chair with your back facing it. Lower yourself down until your glutes touch the chair, then push up to your original standing position. Repeat for 10-15 times.

2. Chair Dips: Firmly grasp the edges of your chair with your hands. Move your feet out in front of you and dip your body down and back up through the strength of your arms. Do this for 10-15 times.

3. Desk Push-Ups: Stand about a meter away from your desk placing your hands on it. Lower your body towards the desk and push back to your original position, doing 10-15 reps.

These are just starter exercises. As you gain strength and confidence, aim to step it up by performing these exercises for longer periods or more repetitions.

4.3. Posture and Flexibility

Maintaining good posture is essential in office environments, it keeps musculoskeletal problems at bay. Complementing this with activities that enhance flexibility can significantly reduce the strain of sedentary work.

1. Spinal Twist: Sitting tall in your chair, rotate your upper body to the right, using the chair for leverage. Hold the position for 15-20 seconds then switch to the left. This will improve spine flexibility and also promote better posture.

2. Chest Opener: Clasp your hands behind your back, straighten your arms and lift your head. Hold for 15 to 20 seconds. Along with bettering your posture, this stretch opens up your chest, aiding in efficient breathing.

These are exercises designed for a tiny office space with the simple aim of helping you transform your sedentary workday into an active one.

4.4. Office Exercise Routine Incorporation

Transitioning from a sedentary to a more active working environment might seem challenging initially; however, making small, incremental changes is more manageable and sustainable. Plan short movement breaks into your workday - this could be between meetings, after finishing a task, or during lunchtime. This shift towards an active routine will not only promote physical health but also boost mental wellbeing, resulting in increased productivity and motivation.

By embracing a wellness-focused mindset, these office-friendly exercises can effortlessly co-exist with your busy schedules. Soon, you will discover that fitness isn't a distant goal but a lifestyle choice that is easily attainable even within the four walls of your workspace.

Remember, every step you take towards wellness becomes a partnership between better health and peak professional productivity. This way, you're not just conquering the chair, but also paving the way towards a balance between work and wellness that ensures a triumphant you both in the boardroom and beyond.

Chapter 5. Healthy Eats: Boosting Metabolism with the Right Foods

Food has a profound impact on our bodies and our mind. What we consume not only gives us energy to go about our daily tasks but also helps to regulate our metabolism, influencing how we digest and metabolize that energy. Finding balance and making conscious decisions about what we fuel our bodies with can lead to significant improvements not just in our physical health but also our mental stamina. Here, we will shed light on foods that are known to boost metabolism, aiding in weight management and overall wellness.

5.1. The science behind metabolism

Metabolism includes all the biochemical processes that take place within our body to maintain life. These processes allow us to grow, reproduce, repair damage, and respond to our environment. It is often divide into two categories:

1. Catabolism: the breakdown of molecules to obtain energy

2. Anabolism: the synthesis of all compounds needed by the cells

The Basal Metabolic Rate (BMR) relates to the number of calories you burn while at rest. Roughly 60-75% of the calories you burn each day are to maintain basic bodily functions like your heartbeat and breathing. Things such as your age, sex, and muscle mass can affect your BMR.

5.2. Metabolism-boosting foods

Several foods have been studied for their potential to increase metabolism or maintain efficient metabolic function. Here are top choices you may want to consider:

1. Protein-rich foods: Consuming protein can increase your metabolic rate by inducing the Thermic Effect of Food (TEF), a phenomenon where the body uses additional calories to digest, absorb, and process nutrients in your meal. Foods high in protein include lean meats, dairy, eggs, and legumes.

2. Green tea: Beyond its host of antioxidants, green tea has been associated with increased fat burning and metabolic rate.

3. Legumes and pulses: Lentils, chickpeas, peas, and beans are high in protein and fiber content, which supports efficient metabolism and feelings of fullness.

4. Whole grains: Foods like oatmeal and brown rice are rich in fiber, requiring more energy to breakdown and digest than processed grains.

5. Chili peppers: Capsaicin, a chemical found in spicy food, can potentially boost your metabolism by increasing the number of calories and fat you burn.

6. Coffee: Known for its caffeine content, coffee can aid in boosting metabolism and promoting fat burning albeit with varied efficacy depending on individual characteristics.

Remember, while these foods can aid in boosting your metabolism, they are not magic bullets for weight loss. Regular exercise, good sleep, and an overall balanced diet are necessary for overall metabolic health.

5.3. Incorporating metabolism boosting foods in your daily diet

Start your day with a metabolism-boosting breakfast. Try a protein-rich option like Greek yogurt with a scoop of almonds and berries or whole grain toast with avocado and eggs. These foods can help rev up your metabolism, keep you feeling full, and provide a burst of energy to start your day right.

For lunch and dinner, aim for a balance of lean protein, fiber-rich vegetables and grains, and healthy fats. Lentil or chickpea salad, grilled chicken with quinoa and steamed vegetables or salmon with brown rice and grilled asparagus are delicious examples of how to combine these elements.

Snacks can be an opportunity to include metabolism-boosting foods too. Try a green tea in the afternoon for a pick-me-up or munch on some chili-lime roasted chickpeas for a savory snack.

Remember to also drink plenty of water throughout the day. Hydration helps your body carry out metabolic processes efficiently.

5.4. Conclusion: Your personal best

Metabolism is a personal thing - what works for one person might not work for another. It's about finding the best balance that supports your body and makes you feel your best. Remember that a diet high in fruits, vegetables, lean proteins, whole grains, and with the right kind of fats is the best approach to a healthy metabolism. And while our focus here has been food, exercise, sleep, and stress management all play critical roles in your overall metabolism too.

Gradually incorporate these suggestions into your daily routine, remember the importance of balance and variety in your diet, and listen to your body's signals. Here's to healthier and happier days at work as you embrace this metabolism-boosting dietary shift!

Chapter 6. Exercise Schedule: Workouts for the Busy Bees

Let's delve into creating an exercise regimen that harmonizes with your hectic workdays. Endlessly packed calendars, impromptu meetings, and tight deadlines do not necessarily equate to an inactive, sedentary lifestyle. In reality, balancing fitness with corporate responsibilities doesn't require a heroic effort, but rather a strategic and manageable approach. The supplied exercise schedule, peppered with a variety of movement types and adapted to your work environment, will ensure that fitness easily slides into your bustling life.

6.1. The Magic of Movement: Why Exercise?

Before we delve into the specifics, let's explore why movement is crucial. Regular exercise provides numerous health benefits, including reducing the risk of developing chronic diseases, improving mood and energy levels, and promoting better sleep. Furthermore, it enhances cognition and productivity levels. A brief workout can refresh your mind, infusing it with clarity and creating an open window for creative ideas. It's clear that making room for exercise is not just about physical health but also enhances your cognitive abilities, ultimately leading to increased performance and efficiency at work.

6.2. Exercise Blueprint for a Week

Here is a one-week exercise blueprint. This schedule is flexible and can be adjusted to your personal commitments, physical abilities, and comfort levels.

NOTE: It's essential to consult your physician before embarking on any new exercise regimen.

Day	Morning (Before Work)	Mid-day (Lunch Break)	Evening (After Work)
Monday	10 min Stretching	Office Chair Yoga (15 min)	20 min Cardio (Dance/Zumba)
Tuesday	10 min Pilates	Staircase Workout (10 min)	20 min Strength Training (Bodyweight/Weights)
Wednesday	10 min Mobility Drills	Desk Push-ups, Tricep Dips (10 min)	30 min Walk/Jog
Thursday	Rest	Walk and Stretch Breaks (10 min)	Rest
Friday	10 min Dynamic Yoga	Desk Exercises (Leg raises, seated twists – 10 min)	30 min Cardio (Skipping/Cycling)
Saturday	Rest	Weekend	Rest
Sunday	Rest	Weekend	Optional Activity (Day off – Opt for something fun like Hiking/Tennis/Swimming)

6.3. Exercises in Detail

Morning Workouts

Morning workouts can provide an energy boost that lasts throughout the day. Starting your day with an exercise routine will not only help you become physically active but also help you clear your mind and prepare for the tasks at hand.

- **Stretching**: An excellent way to wake up your muscles; focus on all the major muscle groups.

- **Pilates**: Builds core strength and improves flexibility. Basic movements can be easily carried out at home.

- **Mobility Drills**: These exercises, such as arm circles and ankle rotations, improve joint mobility.

- **Dynamic Yoga**: Infuses energy and aids in body flexibility and strength.

Mid-day Workouts

Sneaking in short bursts of exercise during your lunch break can be a real game changer. It's not about making huge commitments; instead, it's about utilizing those spare moments to move around.

- **Office Chair Yoga**: Stretches that can be done sitting in your office chair itself; aids with relaxation and posture.

- **Staircase Workout**: Skipping the elevator and taking the stairs; a few rounds can get your heart pumping.

- **Desk Push-ups, Tricep Dips**: Strength-building exercises using your desk or a sturdy chair.

- **Desk Exercises**: Leg raises and seated twists to help tone your muscles.

Evening or After Work Workouts

Unwind after a busy day with a workout that works up a sweat or helps relieve stress.

- **Cardio (Dance/Zumba/ Skipping/Cycling)**: A fun way to get your heart rate up and burn calories.

- **Strength Training (Bodyweight/Weights)**: Work on building muscles and strength; you can start with bodyweight exercises and gradually incorporate weights.

- **Walk/Jog**: Helps clear your mind, unwind, and adds to your daily step count.

Consistent small changes will contribute enormously to your wellness journey. Remember that every step counts, every stretch matters, and consistency is key. So, devise your schedule, prepare your mind, unroll your exercise mat, and set sail on this amazing wellness adventure! Let's convert your 'busy' into 'active' and 'healthy.'

Chapter 7. Superfoods Unveiled: Your Allies for a Healthier Life

Eating right goes hand-in-hand with exercising regularly when it comes to maintaining a healthy lifestyle. In the corporate world, where stress and pressure are inevitable, consuming nutrient-dense foods, also known as superfoods, can make a significant difference to your physical health and mental wellbeing. Superfoods imbued with essential nutrients help to boost your energy, improve brain function, and reduce the risk of chronic diseases. Let's explore these superfoods in greater depth.

7.1. Understanding Superfoods

Superfoods are nutritionally dense, meaning they offer more nutrients — vitamins, minerals, antioxidants, fiber, and others — relative to their calorie content compared to other types of food. These foods can be fruits, vegetables, nuts, seeds, and even fish or lean meats. Superfoods don't have a scientific or standard definition; it's more of a marketing term. However, these foods are undeniably healthy and beneficial for the overall wellness of your body and mind.

While superfoods offer several health benefits, it's worth remembering that no single food or food group can offer all the nutrition you need. Superfoods can supplement a balanced diet, but they aren't a quick fix or miracle cure.

7.2. Boost Your Day with These Superfoods

Here's a list of a few essential superfoods that you can easily incorporate into your regular diet.

7.2.1. Berries

Berries, including blueberries, strawberries, raspberries, and blackberries, are packed with vitamins, fiber, and antioxidants. They can contribute to your daily fruit intake and make for a handy snack when you're feeling peckish between meals.

7.2.2. Nuts and Seeds

Nuts, like almonds and walnuts, and seeds including chia seeds and flaxseeds, are high in fiber, healthy fats, and vitamins. They can be eaten raw, roasted, or blended into a smoothie. But, beware of their high calorie count, moderation is key here.

7.2.3. Whole Grains

Whole grains such as oats, brown rice, and quinoa provide a slow-release energy source that keeps you full for longer. They also contain fiber along with several other nutrients.

7.2.4. Leafy Green Vegetables

Leafy greens, such as spinach and kale, are high in fiber and rich in vitamins A, C, and K, and other nutrients. Incorporating more of these into your diet could help protect against chronic illnesses like heart disease and diabetes.

7.2.5. Fatty Fish

Fatty fish like salmon, mackerel, and sardines are rich in Omega-3 fatty acids that are known to promote heart health and improve mental function.

7.2.6. Avocados

Avocados are high in healthy fats, fibers, and several vitamins. They're also an excellent source of the antioxidant lutein, which is important for eye health.

7.3. Incorporating Superfoods in Your Daily Diet

So, how can you include these nutrient powerhouses in your daily diet, particularly when you're in a busy corporate world? Here are a few suggestions.

7.3.1. Plan Your Meals

Planning your meals in advance can make a huge difference. This way, you know you'll be packing in the nutrients, even if your day gets unexpectedly busy. Make a list, stick it on your fridge, and use it to guide your grocery shopping.

7.3.2. Prepare Smoothies

Combined the right way, smoothies can be superfood powerhouses. For instance, blend a portion of leafy greens with mixed berries and a spoonful of chia seeds for an antioxidant-rich smoothie that's great for breakfast or a mid-afternoon snack.

7.3.3. Snack Smart

Swap your regular snacks with superfood alternatives. Instead of reaching out for a chocolate bar when your energy dips, snack on a handful of nuts or a piece of dark chocolate, which is high in antioxidants.

7.4. Why Metabolism Matters

Metabolism refers to all the chemical reactions in your body that maintain your living state. In simpler terms, it's the process of converting the food you eat into the energy your body uses. A healthy metabolism is crucial for energy, managing weight, and overall wellness. And the good news? You can boost your metabolism with certain superfoods!

7.4.1. Green Tea

Green tea is loaded with antioxidants and a potent compound known as epigallocatechin gallate (EGCG). EGCG has been shown to boost metabolism and promote weight loss.

7.4.2. Spices

Including spices like ginger, cinnamon, and chilli peppers in your meals can not only enhance the flavor but also increase metabolic rate.

7.4.3. Beans and Legumes

Beans and legumes are rich in protein, which requires more energy to digest, therefore boosting your metabolism.

7.4.4. Water

Though not typically classified as a superfood, water is crucial to bodily functions, including metabolism. Dehydration can reduce metabolic function, so ensure you're drinking plenty of water each day.

7.5. Conclusion

The term "superfood" may be a marketing gimmick, but there's no denying the health benefits of these nutrient-rich foods. They're packed with essential vitamins, minerals, and antioxidants that do wonders for your body and mind, especially if you're navigating a busy corporate lifestyle. But remember, maintaining a balanced diet is key. No single food can offer all the nutrition your body needs. Aim for a colorful plate with a variety of foods, and reap the health and wellness benefits.

Chapter 8. The Art of Mindful Eating in a Corporate Environment

Eating mindfully means being fully present for what you're doing while you're doing it and that includes the act of nourishing your body with food. It's about recognizing and respecting your body's hunger and fullness cues, enjoying the taste, texture, and aroma of your food, and being aware of how your eating habits affect your wellbeing. In a corporate environment, where stress and busyness often make it difficult to focus, it's especially important to cultivate this practice.

8.1. Understanding Mindful Eating

Let's first delve into the understanding of mindful eating. Simply put, mindful eating, derived from the Buddhist concept of mindfulness, is a practice that encourages being fully present and engaged in the eating experience. It's a break away from distracted or emotional eating and focuses more on cultivating an understanding between you, your food, and your body's needs.

Mindful eating is not a diet or a quick fix; rather, it's an ongoing journey of exploring food, hunger, and satisfaction. It helps individuals develop a balanced, respectful, healthy, and joyful relationship with food and eating, beneficial for physical and mental health.

8.2. The Relevance of Mindful Eating in a Corporate Setting

In the hustle-bustle of the business world, you often eat meals at your desk, during meetings, or on the way to a meeting. This type of unconscious, distracted eating may lead to overeating, digestion problems, and ultimately weight gain and reduced wellness.

Mindful eating acts as a counter to this fast-paced eating habit. It encourages you to take the time to prepare your food, sit down away from your desk, and focus on eating. This not only aids digestion but may improve your relationship with food, reduce overeating, and promote better overall health.

8.3. Practical Ways to Bring Mindfulness to Your Meals

Now, let's explore some practical ways of incorporating mindful eating into your workday.

Firstly, honor your body's hunger and fullness cues. Try to eat when you're moderately hungry and stop when you're comfortably full, rather than waiting until you're starving or eating until you're stuffed. This suppresses overeating and under-eating.

Secondly, eat without distractions. It's easy to lose track of how much you're eating when you're working, scrolling through social media, or watching TV. Set a time for meals where you can focus on eating.

Also, savor your food. Take the time to chew thoroughly and notice the taste, texture, and aroma of each bite. This makes eating more pleasurable and can help you feel more satisfied with smaller portions.

Lastly, cultivate gratitude for your food. Consider the work that went into producing, distributing, and preparing the food you eat. This helps promote a positive relationship with food.

8.4. Mindful Eating Exercises for the Workplace

Practice these exercises to help hone mindful eating skills:

1. *Buddy lunches*: Schedule lunches with colleagues where everyone focuses on eating. Share perceptions of taste, texture, and aroma.

2. *Mindful snacking*: Keep a personal stash of tasty, healthy snacks. When hunger strikes, find a quiet place, and eat your snack slowly, savoring each bite.

3. *Mindful breathing*: Before you eat, take a few moments to breathe deeply and relax your body. This can help prime your body for better digestion and help you focus on your meal.

8.5. Foods That Promote Mindfulness

Certain foods naturally promote mindfulness and should be incorporated into your diet. These include:

- *Complex carbohydrates* like whole grains and legumes, which provide steady energy and keep you satiated longer.

- *Healthy fats* like avocados and nuts, which keep you full and support overall health.

- *Fruits and vegetables*, which are packed with essential nutrients and can help improve concentration and overall health.

- *Probiotic-rich foods* like yogurt, which promote a healthy gut and can improve mental health.

To wrap up, mindful eating is a multifaceted practice, especially suitable for the corporate environment, that emphasizes active engagement during the process of eating, from choosing your food to savouring every bite. In practice, it requires incorporating mindful eating techniques, practicing exercises that promote mindfulness, and selecting foods that naturally stimulate mindfulness. By integrating mindful eating, you can nourish your body and mind while improving your relationship with food for better work-life health balance.

Chapter 9. Success Stories: Transformations within the Workplace

In the challenging landscape of corporate health, a number of companies have emerged as torchbearers of transformation. They've turned company culture on its head – creating healthier, happier environments for their employees, and in the process, redefined the idea of a productive workplace. Let us delve into some inspiring transformation narratives within the workplace.

9.1. Company One: Tech Giants Embrace Wellness

In the heart of Silicon Valley, one tech titan has prioritized wellness alongside innovation. Realizing that the best output comes from well-rested, well-nurtured minds, they implemented a holistic wellness approach - creating spaces within their campus for physical fitness, mental relaxation, and healthy eating.

Indoor fitness centers with state-of-the-art equipment became commonplace, staffed by certified trainers, and complemented by wellness programs such as yoga and Zumba classes. Comfortable, tech-free zones were introduced - havens for employees to momentarily disconnect and recharge. Conscious effort was made to transform the cafeteria, offering a range of whole foods, locally sourced and cooked fresh.

Their efforts bore fruitful results. Employees reported increased morale, reduced stress, and enhanced productivity. Absenteeism was slashed, and talent retention skyrocketed. Subscriptions to wellness programs signified a wider acceptance of the healthy shift in culture.

9.2. Company Two: Transition to a Health-conscious Culture

A multinational retail giant embarked on a determined journey towards a healthier corporate environment. Initially plagued by frequent sick leaves, high employee turnover and dilating healthcare costs, the company took firm steps to introduce wholesale changes in their approach towards employee wellness.

The company introduced standing desks, ergonomically designed workstations, and regular fitness challenges. Break times were incentivized for short, brisk walks. The canteen menu saw an overhaul, replacing processed foods with healthier alternatives. Water coolers amplified conversations on wellness and healthy habits.

Within a year, the company registered a noticeable decline in sick leave applications and related costs. Employees reported feeling happier, more energized and valued. The cumulative effect was seen in better customer service, increased sales, and stronger rapport among team members.

9.3. Company Three: Financial Firm's Healthy Investment

A globally recognized financial services company recognized the detriments of employee burnouts and adopted a proactive approach to protect and promote employee health.

They launched a dedicated wellness portal, offering online resources for physical and mental health, including guides for home workouts, stress management techniques and dietary tips. Regular interactive webinars featured health and fitness professionals providing expert advice. The firm offered partial reimbursement of gym membership fees, encouraging employees to actively participate in regular exercise.

The firm saw a significant dip in health care costs and employee absenteeism. The firm's investment in wellness paid off with improved employee morale, higher productivity and an overall increase in employee satisfaction.

These success stories signify a paradigm shift in corporate culture, fostering the belief that employee wellness isn't just an optional extra but a core part of a thriving business. Indeed, companies that have invested in the wellbeing of their staff have seen tangible benefits in retained talent, boosted morale, and enhanced productivity. Most importantly, such companies have brought about a meaningful transformation, empowering their employees to lead better, healthier lives, both within and outside the workplace. As these companies have demonstrated, workplace transformations are not just possible, they're profitable too.

Chapter 10. Tools and Apps: Tech Support for Corporate Wellness

In an exciting era marked by rapid technology advancement, health and wellness are no longer being left behind. There are a multitude of digital tools and applications available to aid any health-conscious corporate employee in achieving their wellness goals. Whether you need assistance with healthy office workouts, staying hydrated, or managing stress, there's an app for it! These tools are tremendously versatile, catering to a diverse range of needs while ensuring the maintenance of a healthy work-life balance.

10.1. Office Fitness Apps

Office fitness apps are your digital fitness trainers, available at your fingertips. They provide office-appropriate exercises that can be completed sitting at your desk, before a meeting, or in a short break. They guide you in maintaining physical activity without disrupting your workflow.

1. *7 Minute Workout: Fitness App* This app offers exercise routines that can be completed in just seven minutes, making it perfect for a quick office break, without the need for specialized gym equipment. Not only will these exercises help you stay physically fit, they're also great for re-energizing and increasing productivity.

2. *Office Workout & Fitness* Offers a comprehensive collection of exercises intended to be office-friendly. It includes exercises for different body parts, allowing you to focus on specific areas and prevent problems caused by prolonged sitting, like stiff neck, back pain, and poor circulation.

3. ***Stand Up! The Work Break Timer*** The Stand Up! app offers a subtle reminder for office workers to stand, stretch, and avoid prolonged periods of sitting. You can set your schedules based on your working hours and break frequency, helping you maintain a healthy office lifestyle.

10.2. Health and Nutritional Apps

Proper nutrition is critical for maintaining our overall wellbeing. These designated apps are equipped to assist you with healthy food choices and nutrient tracking to keep metabolism running smoothly.

1. ***MyFitnessPal*** This app provides comprehensive nutritional information about various food items. It allows you to track your daily calorie intake and offers wellness tips, making it easier for you to achieve your dietary goals and better manage your weight.

2. ***Water Drink Reminder*** Staying hydrated is an overlooked yet vital part of maintaining good health. This app reminds you to drink water throughout the day and allows you to monitor your daily water intake, contributing positively to your wellness crusade.

10.3. Mental Wellness Apps

Mental wellbeing is an integral part of overall health, and there's a plethora of apps catering to various aspects like stress management, meditation, sleep improvement, etc.

1. ***Headspace*** Headspace offers guided meditations crafted to assist in stress management, focus improvement, and sleep enhancement. These practices contribute significantly to mental wellbeing, making the app a must-have in the corporate wellness toolbox.

2. ***Calm*** The app offers numerous mindfulness exercises and sleep

aid stories along with relaxing music tracks which can help manage the stress of a busy workday, ensuring proper mental relaxation.

10.4. Posture Improvement Apps

Correct posture is a vital yet frequently disregarded element of corporate wellness. Many health issues arise due to improper posture owing to prolonged sitting.

1. ***Posture Reminder*** This app offers posture correction exercises and sends reminders to check your posture. This can significantly help in reducing strain on your back and neck, promoting better body alignment.

2. ***Upright GO Posture Trainer*** It's a wearable device that vibrates when you slouch, encouraging you to straighten up. The linked app helps you track your progress over time, leading to lasting posture improvement.

In conclusion, these tools and apps provide easily accessible support for corporate wellness. It's no surprise that incorporating these technological aids into your routine can significantly improve your physical fitness, nutritional habits, mental wellness, and posture. It's crucial to remember, though, to select the tools that best suit your personal needs and preferences. Begin experimenting with these tech tools, make informed choices, and start your journey towards wellness today!

Chapter 11. Charting the Future: Sustaining Wellness in a Corporate World

The pursuit of wellness in a corporate world is not a short-lived trend, rather it is a paradigm shift towards a more holistic approach to work-life balance. As the urgency of mental and physical health takes center stage, this shift becomes an essential aspect in shaping the future of the corporate world. Here's an in-depth look at sustaining wellness in a corporate environment.

11.1. Embracing the Wellness Culture

To attain and sustain wellness, it's essential to group it into two categories: physical health and mental wellbeing. On the physical side, regular exercise and nutrition significantly contribute to maintaining a healthy body. For mental health, an environment that promotes peacefulness, creativity, and reduces stress plays a significant role.

However, consistently incorporating these health measures requires more than a personal commitment. An organization should cultivate a wellness culture that makes these practices more accessible to employees, and integrates wellness into the broader corporate ethos. Such a culture not only boosts morale and productivity but also reduces burnout while increasing staff retention.

11.2. Health and Wellness Programs

Wellness programs that offer guidance on nutrition, exercise, and mental health can become a cornerstone in fostering this culture. Regular health checkups, mental health seminars, gym memberships, yoga classes, and nutrition counselling are some features that organizations can explore.

However, these initiatives ought to be tailored to the requirements of the employees. Regular feedback and quantifiable insights can ensure that wellness programs are both effective and popular.

11.3. Workspace Redesign

Sometimes, the workspace itself can be a deterrent or a motivator for wellness. Open layouts that invite natural light, areas designated for relaxation, and physical amenities such as exercise tools can revolutionize workspace wellness. Even simple directives like standing desks or ergonomically designed office furniture can significantly impact an employees' physical well-being.

11.4. Flexibility and Work-Life Balance

Flexibility has gained newfound importance in the pursuit of work-life balance. What primarily matters is the task completion rather than where the tasks are being done. Hence, flexible timings can give employees the leisure to attend their wellness needs without overlapping their work schedule. Additionally, providing a remote work arrangement can help employees cut back on commute stress, give them more time for personal work, and increase productivity.

11.5. Investing in Technology

Numerous wellness applications and wearable devices today provide features ranging from sleep tracking to nutrition logging. Investing in such technologies can ease the way employees track their health statistics and goals, making them feel more in control of their own wellness.

11.6. Mental Health Support

On par with physical wellness, mental health must be addressed comprehensively. Encouraging open conversations about stress and mental health can help eliminate the taboo that often surrounds it. Offering mental health resources—such as counseling services—and incorporating mindfulness or stress-management techniques into the workday can significantly contribute to employee wellness.

11.7. Participation and Incentives

To encourage participation in wellness programs, companies must provide attractive incentives. These could range from health insurance benefits to acknowledging the 'healthiest' department or individual.

In the end, the efficacy of these initiatives lies in their execution. While variety might attract some, others might appreciate simplicity. As an organization, it's crucial to continually evolve and adapt to the needs and preferences of the employees. This ensures that wellness becomes an ongoing journey towards better health, better productivity, and a better corporate culture.

Envisioning a future that places employee wellness at its core may seem like a daunting task. Still, with calculated steps and deliberate strategies, it is more than achievable. After all, a well and happy employee is an asset beyond measure. So, let's press on and continue to chart this exciting future together!

11.8. Conclusion

The journey to a future where wellness is a priority within the corporate world is one full of obstacles and opportunities. As the needs and requirements of the employees are continually evolving, organizations must adapt their wellness policies and work environment to meet those demands.

In the end, it all boils down to this simple truth — a healthy employee is a happy employee, and a happy employee is a productive one. With focused intent, consistent efforts, and a deep understanding of the wellness needs of its employees, an organization can effectively foster an environment that promotes and sustains wellness in the corporate world.

So let's start today, move forward with purpose and conscious effort to make wellness a mainstay in our workplaces. Each step we take in this direction is a guaranteed investment for the future — a future teeming with wellness, productivity, and prosperity.